Zero Point Wonders: The Ultimate Weight Loss Cookbook.

Simple, Tasty Recipes for a Healthier Lifestyle

Victor C. Sell

Copyright©2024 Victor C. Sell

All right reserved. No part of this publication may be reproduced, distributed, or transmitted in any form or by any means, including photocopying, recording, or other electronic or mechanical methods, without the prior written permission of the publisher, except in the case of brief quotation embodied in critical reviews and certain other noncommercial uses permitted by copyright law.

Contents

1. Introduction
- Overview of zero-point foods
- Benefits of a zero-point diet for weight loss and overall health

2. Breakfast Boosters
- Quick and nutritious zero-point breakfast ideas
- Recipes: Smoothie Bowls, Veggie Omelets, Fruit Salads

3. Mid-Morning Snacks
- Healthy snack options to keep you energized
- Recipes: Apple Slices with Cinnamon, Veggie Sticks with Hummus

4. Lunch Lightness
- Filling yet light zero-point lunch recipes
- Recipes: Zesty Quinoa Salad, Grilled Chicken Lettuce Wraps

5. Afternoon Pick-Me-Ups
- Snacks to beat the afternoon slump
- Recipes: Greek Yogurt with Berries, Air-Popped Popcorn

6. Dinner Delights
- Delicious and satisfying zero-point dinner ideas
- Recipes: Baked Lemon Herb Fish, Spaghetti Squash with Tomato Sauce

7. Sweet Treats
- Indulgent yet guilt-free desserts
- Recipes: Frozen Fruit Sorbet, Baked Cinnamon Apples

8. Hydration Heroes
- Zero-point drinks and smoothies to stay hydrated
- Recipes: Cucumber Mint Water, Green Detox Smoothie.

9. Party Pleasers
- Zero-point appetizers and party snacks
- Recipes: Shrimp Cocktail, Stuffed Mushrooms

10. Meal Prepping Made Easy
- Tips for planning and preparing zero-point meals ahead of time
- Recipes: Batch Cooking Veggie Soup, Overnight Oats

11. On-the-Go Options
- Portable zero-point snacks and meals
- Recipes: Mason Jar Salads, Protein-Packed Snack Bars

12. Kid-Friendly Favorites
- Zero-point recipes that kids will love
- Recipes: Mini Veggie Pizzas, Banana Ice Cream

13. Cultural Cuisine
- Zero-point recipes inspired by global flavors

- Recipes: Mexican Cauliflower Rice, Thai Cucumber Salad

14. Comfort Food Classics
- Zero-point versions of beloved comfort foods
- Recipes: Cauliflower Mac and Cheese, Turkey Chili

15. Fitness Fuel
- Zero-point recipes to support an active lifestyle
- Recipes: Power Protein Pancakes, Post-Workout Smoothies

16. Budget-Friendly Bites
- Economical zero-point meal ideas
- Recipes: Lentil Stew, Chickpea Salad

17. Holiday and Special Occasion Recipes
- Zero-point recipes for festive occasions
- Recipes: Holiday Veggie Platter, Summer Berry Parfait

18. Time-Saving Tips
- Quick and easy zero-point recipes for busy days
- Recipes: Instant Pot Chicken Soup, Microwave Steamed Veggies

19. Mindful Eating
- Strategies for enjoying zero-point foods mindfully
- Recipes: Slow-Cooked Ratatouille, Savor-the-Moment Salad

20. Conclusion
- Recap of the benefits of zero-point eating
- Encouragement to continue the journey towards a healthier lifestyle

Introduction: Overview of Zero-Point Foods, Benefits of a Zero-Point Diet for Weight Loss and Overall Health

Welcome to "Zero Point Wonders: The Ultimate Weight Loss Cookbook: Simple, Tasty Recipes for a Healthier Lifestyle." This book is your guide to a revolutionary way of eating that focuses on zero-point foods—nutritious, satisfying, and versatile ingredients that can help you achieve and maintain a healthier lifestyle without the stress of counting calories or points.

What Are Zero-Point Foods?

Zero-point foods are those that you can eat freely without having to measure or track them. These foods are typically nutrient-dense, low in calories, and high in essential vitamins and minerals. They include a wide variety of fruits, vegetables, lean proteins, and certain grains and legumes. The concept of zero-point foods is designed to simplify your eating habits, making it easier to maintain a balanced diet and achieve your weight loss goals.

The Benefits of a Zero-Point Diet

1. Weight Loss: By focusing on zero-point foods, you naturally reduce your calorie intake without feeling deprived. These foods are filling and satisfying, which helps control hunger and prevent overeating.

2. Nutritional Balance: Zero-point foods are packed with essential nutrients, ensuring that your body gets the vitamins, minerals, and antioxidants it needs to function optimally. This promotes overall health and well-being.

3. Simplicity: One of the biggest advantages of a zero-point diet is its simplicity. There's no need to meticulously count calories or points for every meal. Instead, you can enjoy a wide variety of foods without the stress of constant tracking.

4. Sustainability: Because zero-point foods are typically whole, unprocessed, and naturally low in calories, they form the foundation of a sustainable eating plan. This means you can stick to this way of eating long-term, making it easier to maintain your weight loss.

5. Improved Digestion: Many zero-point foods are rich in fiber, which aids in digestion and helps keep your digestive system healthy. Fiber also contributes to feelings of fullness, further supporting weight management.

6. Increased Energy Levels: Eating a diet rich in zero-point foods can boost your energy levels. These foods provide steady, sustained energy, helping you feel more vibrant and active throughout the day.

7. Better Blood Sugar Control: Zero-point foods, particularly those high in fiber and protein, can help stabilize blood sugar levels. This is especially beneficial for those managing diabetes or trying to prevent blood sugar spikes and crashes.

8. Heart Health: Many zero-point foods, such as fruits, vegetables, and lean proteins, are heart-healthy. They can help reduce cholesterol levels, lower blood pressure, and decrease the risk of heart disease.

In this book, you will find an array of delicious and simple recipes that showcase the versatility and flavor of zero-point foods. From breakfast boosters to dinner delights, each recipe is designed to support your weight loss journey while keeping your taste buds satisfied. Alongside the recipes, you'll find practical tips and strategies for incorporating zero-point foods into your daily life, ensuring that you can enjoy a healthier, happier lifestyle with ease.

Embark on this journey with us and discover the wonders of zero-point eating. Your path to a healthier, more vibrant you starts here.

Breakfast Boosters: Quick and Nutritious Zero-Point Breakfast Ideas

Starting your day with a nutritious breakfast is essential for maintaining energy levels, supporting metabolism, and setting a positive tone for the rest of your day. Here are ten zero-point breakfast recipes that are both delicious and easy to prepare. From smoothie bowls to veggie omelets and fruit salads, these recipes will help you kickstart your day on a healthy note.

1. Berry Bliss Smoothie Bowl

***Ingredients*:**
- 1 cup mixed berries (strawberries, blueberries, raspberries)
- 1 banana
- 1 cup unsweetened almond milk
- 1 tablespoon chia seeds
- 1 tablespoon unsweetened shredded coconut

Instructions:

1. Blend the mixed berries, banana, and almond milk until smooth.
2. Pour the smoothie into a bowl.
3. Top with chia seeds and shredded coconut.
4. Enjoy immediately.

2. Tropical Paradise Smoothie Bowl

Ingredients:
- 1 cup pineapple chunks
- 1 mango, peeled and chopped
- 1 banana
- 1 cup coconut water
- 1 tablespoon ground flaxseed

Instructions:

1. Blend the pineapple, mango, banana, and coconut water until smooth.
2. Pour the smoothie into a bowl.
3. Sprinkle with ground flaxseed.
4. Serve immediately.

3. Green Power Smoothie Bowl
Ingredients:
- 1 cup spinach
- 1 kiwi, peeled and chopped
- 1 banana
- 1/2 cup unsweetened almond milk
- 1 tablespoon chia seeds

Instructions:

1. Blend the spinach, kiwi, banana, and almond milk until smooth.
2. Pour the smoothie into a bowl.
3. Top with chia seeds.
4. Serve immediately.

4. Veggie Omelet

Ingredients:
- 1/2 cup chopped bell peppers (red, green, yellow)
- 1/2 cup chopped onions
- 1/2 cup chopped mushrooms
- 1/2 cup spinach
- 2 large eggs

- Salt and pepper to taste

Instructions:

1. In a non-stick skillet, sauté the bell peppers, onions, and mushrooms until tender.
2. Add the spinach and cook until wilted.
3. Whisk the eggs with salt and pepper and pour over the veggies.
4. Cook until the eggs are set.
5. Fold the omelet and serve immediately.

5. Tomato Basil Veggie Omelet

Ingredients:
- 1/2 cup cherry tomatoes, halved
- 1/4 cup fresh basil, chopped
- 1/2 cup chopped zucchini
- 2 large eggs
- Salt and pepper to taste

Instructions:

1. In a non-stick skillet, sauté the tomatoes and zucchini until tender.

2. Add the basil and cook for an additional minute.
3. Whisk the eggs with salt and pepper and pour over the veggies.
4. Cook until the eggs are set.
5. Fold the omelet and serve immediately.

6. Classic Fruit Salad

Ingredients:
- 1 apple, chopped
- 1 banana, sliced
- 1 cup grapes, halved
- 1 orange, peeled and segmented
- 1 cup strawberries, sliced

Instructions:
1. In a large bowl, combine all the fruits.
2. Toss gently to mix.
3. Serve immediately or chill until ready to eat.

7. Citrus Berry Fruit Salad

Ingredients:
- 1 grapefruit, peeled and segmented
- 1 orange, peeled and segmented
- 1 cup blueberries
- 1 cup raspberries
- 1 tablespoon fresh mint, chopped

Instructions:
1. In a large bowl, combine the grapefruit, orange, blueberries, and raspberries.
2. Sprinkle with fresh mint and toss gently to mix.
3. Serve immediately or chill until ready to eat.

8. Spiced Apple Smoothie Bowl

Ingredients:
- 1 apple, peeled and chopped
- 1 banana
- 1/2 teaspoon cinnamon
- 1 cup unsweetened almond milk
- 1 tablespoon almond butter

Instructions:

1. Blend the apple, banana, cinnamon, almond milk, and almond butter until smooth.
2. Pour the smoothie into a bowl.
3. Serve immediately.

9. Mediterranean Veggie Omelet

Ingredients:
- 1/2 cup chopped tomatoes
- 1/4 cup chopped olives
- 1/2 cup chopped spinach
- 2 large eggs
- Salt and pepper to taste

Instructions:

1. In a non-stick skillet, sauté the tomatoes, olives, and spinach until tender.
2. Whisk the eggs with salt and pepper and pour over the veggies.
3. Cook until the eggs are set.
4. Fold the omelet and serve immediately.

10. Melon Mint Fruit Salad

Ingredients:
- 1 cup watermelon, cubed
- 1 cup cantaloupe, cubed
- 1 cup honeydew, cubed
- 1 tablespoon fresh mint, chopped

Instructions:
1. In a large bowl, combine the watermelon, cantaloupe, and honeydew.
2. Sprinkle with fresh mint and toss gently to mix.
3. Serve immediately or chill until ready to eat.

Enjoy these quick and nutritious zero-point breakfast ideas that will not only keep you satisfied but also support your weight loss journey.

Mid-Morning Snacks: Healthy Snack Options to Keep You Energized

Mid-morning snacks can be crucial for maintaining energy levels and preventing overeating at lunchtime. These zero-point snacks are not only healthy but also easy to prepare, ensuring you stay on track with your weight loss goals. Here are five delicious and nutritious recipes to enjoy:

1. Apple Slices with Cinnamon

***Ingredients*:**
- 1 apple, sliced
- 1/2 teaspoon ground cinnamon

***Instructions*:**
1. Wash and core the apple, then cut it into thin slices.
2. Arrange the apple slices on a plate.
3. Sprinkle ground cinnamon evenly over the apple slices.

4. Serve immediately for a sweet and satisfying snack.

2. Veggie Sticks with Hummus

Ingredients:
- 1 carrot, cut into sticks
- 1 cucumber, cut into sticks
- 1 bell pepper, cut into sticks
- 1/2 cup cherry tomatoes
- 1/2 cup homemade hummus

Instructions:
1. Wash and cut the vegetables into sticks.
2. Arrange the veggie sticks and cherry tomatoes on a plate.
3. Serve with a side of homemade hummus for dipping.

Homemade Hummus Recipe:

- 1 can chickpeas, drained and rinsed
- 1 garlic clove, minced
- 2 tablespoons lemon juice

- 2 tablespoons tahini
- 1/4 teaspoon ground cumin
- Salt to taste
- Water as needed

1. Combine all ingredients in a food processor.
2. Blend until smooth, adding water as needed to reach desired consistency.
3. Serve immediately or store in the refrigerator.

3. Greek Yogurt with Berries

Ingredients:
- 1 cup non-fat Greek yogurt
- 1/2 cup mixed berries (strawberries, blueberries, raspberries)
- 1 teaspoon honey (optional)

Instructions:
1. Place the Greek yogurt in a bowl.
2. Top with mixed berries.
3. Drizzle with honey, if desired.
4. Serve immediately for a protein-packed snack.

4. Air-Popped Popcorn

Ingredients:
- 1/4 cup popcorn kernels
- Salt to taste

Instructions:
1. Place the popcorn kernels in an air popper and pop according to the manufacturer's instructions.
2. Transfer the popped popcorn to a large bowl.
3. Lightly season with salt.
4. Serve immediately for a crunchy, low-calorie snack.

5. Cucumber and Avocado Bites

Ingredients:
- 1 cucumber, sliced into rounds
- 1 avocado, mashed
- 1 tablespoon lemon juice
- Salt and pepper to taste
- Fresh dill for garnish (optional).

Instructions:
1. In a small bowl, mash the avocado with lemon juice, salt, and pepper.
2. Place the cucumber rounds on a serving plate.
3. Top each cucumber round with a spoonful of mashed avocado.
4. Garnish with fresh dill, if desired.
5. Serve immediately for a refreshing and creamy snack.

These mid-morning snacks are designed to keep you energized and satisfied throughout the day while staying within your zero-point food guidelines. Enjoy these healthy options as part of your journey to a healthier lifestyle.

Lunch Lightness: Filling Yet Light Zero-Point Lunch Recipes

Lunchtime is an opportunity to refuel and recharge with meals that are both satisfying and light. These zero-point lunch recipes are designed to keep you full and energized without weighing you down. Here are five delicious recipes, including Zesty Quinoa Salad and Grilled Chicken Lettuce Wraps, to enjoy:

1. Zesty Quinoa Salad

Ingredients:
- 1 cup cooked quinoa
- 1 cup cherry tomatoes, halved
- 1 cucumber, diced
- 1/4 cup red onion, finely chopped
- 1/4 cup fresh parsley, chopped
- 1/4 cup fresh mint, chopped
- Juice of 1 lemon
- 1 tablespoon olive oil (optional)
- Salt and pepper to taste

Instructions:
1. In a large bowl, combine the cooked quinoa, cherry tomatoes, cucumber, red onion, parsley, and mint.
2. Drizzle with lemon juice and olive oil, if using.
3. Season with salt and pepper to taste.

4. Toss well to combine.
5. Serve immediately or chill until ready to eat.

2. Grilled Chicken Lettuce Wraps

Ingredients:
- 2 boneless, skinless chicken breasts
- 1 tablespoon olive oil
- 1 tablespoon soy sauce (low sodium)
- 1 tablespoon lemon juice
- 1 garlic clove, minced
- 1 head of butter lettuce, leaves separated
- 1 carrot, shredded
- 1 cucumber, julienned
- Fresh cilantro, for garnish

Instructions:
1. In a bowl, mix olive oil, soy sauce, lemon juice, and minced garlic.
2. Marinate the chicken breasts in the mixture for at least 30 minutes.
3. Grill the chicken breasts over medium heat until fully cooked, about 6-8 minutes per side.
4. Let the chicken cool slightly, then slice thinly.

5. To assemble the wraps, place chicken slices, shredded carrot, and julienned cucumber on each lettuce leaf.
6. Garnish with fresh cilantro.
7. Serve immediately.

3. Mediterranean Chickpea Salad

Ingredients:
- 1 can chickpeas, drained and rinsed
- 1 cup cherry tomatoes, halved
- 1 cucumber, diced
- 1/4 cup red onion, finely chopped
- 1/4 cup Kalamata olives, sliced
- 1/4 cup feta cheese, crumbled (optional)
- 2 tablespoons fresh parsley, chopped
- Juice of 1 lemon
- 1 tablespoon olive oil (optional)
- Salt and pepper to taste

Instructions:
1. In a large bowl, combine chickpeas, cherry tomatoes, cucumber, red onion, olives, and parsley.

2. Drizzle with lemon juice and olive oil, if using.
3. Season with salt and pepper to taste.
4. Toss well to combine.
5. Serve immediately or chill until ready to eat.

4. Veggie-Stuffed Bell Peppers

Ingredients:
- 4 bell peppers, halved and seeds removed
- 1 cup cooked quinoa
- 1 cup black beans, drained and rinsed
- 1 cup corn kernels
- 1 cup diced tomatoes
- 1/4 cup red onion, finely chopped
- 1/4 cup fresh cilantro, chopped
- 1 teaspoon cumin
- 1 teaspoon chili powder
- Salt and pepper to taste.

Instructions:
1. Preheat oven to 375°F (190°C).
2. In a large bowl, mix cooked quinoa, black beans, corn, diced tomatoes, red onion, cilantro, cumin, chili powder, salt, and pepper.
3. Stuff the bell pepper halves with the quinoa mixture.
4. Place the stuffed peppers in a baking dish.
5. Cover with foil and bake for 25-30 minutes, until the peppers are tender.
6. Serve immediately.

5. Asian Cabbage Salad

Ingredients:
- 4 cups shredded cabbage
- 1 cup shredded carrots
- 1 red bell pepper, thinly sliced
- 1/4 cup fresh cilantro, chopped
- 1/4 cup green onions, chopped
- 2 tablespoons rice vinegar
- 1 tablespoon soy sauce (low sodium)
- 1 tablespoon sesame oil (optional)
- 1 teaspoon honey (optional)

- 1 tablespoon sesame seeds

Instructions:
1. In a large bowl, combine shredded cabbage, carrots, bell pepper, cilantro, and green onions.
2. In a small bowl, whisk together rice vinegar, soy sauce, sesame oil, and honey.
3. Pour the dressing over the salad and toss well to combine.
4. Sprinkle with sesame seeds.
5. Serve immediately or chill until ready to eat.

These filling yet light zero-point lunch recipes will keep you energized and satisfied, making it easier to stay on track with your healthy lifestyle. Enjoy these delicious meals as part of your journey to better health.

Afternoon Pick-Me-Ups: Snacks to Beat the Afternoon Slump

The mid-afternoon slump can be a challenging time to stay focused and energized. These zero-point snacks are perfect for giving you a boost without adding extra calories. Here are five delicious and nutritious recipes to keep you going:

1. Greek Yogurt with Berries

Ingredients:
- 1 cup non-fat Greek yogurt
- 1/2 cup mixed berries (strawberries, blueberries, raspberries)
- 1 teaspoon honey (optional)

Instructions:
1. Place the Greek yogurt in a bowl.
2. Top with mixed berries.
3. Drizzle with honey, if desired.
4. Serve immediately for a protein-packed snack.

2. Air-Popped Popcorn

Ingredients:
- 1/4 cup popcorn kernels
- Salt to taste

Instructions:
1. Place the popcorn kernels in an air popper and pop according to the manufacturer's instructions.
2. Transfer the popped popcorn to a large bowl.
3. Lightly season with salt.
4. Serve immediately for a crunchy, low-calorie snack.

3. Carrot and Cucumber Sticks with Salsa

Ingredients:
- 2 carrots, peeled and cut into sticks
- 1 cucumber, cut into sticks
- 1 cup fresh salsa

Instructions:
1. Wash and cut the carrots and cucumber into sticks.
2. Arrange the veggie sticks on a plate.
3. Serve with a side of fresh salsa for dipping.
4. Enjoy immediately.

4. Edamame with Sea Salt

Ingredients:
- 1 cup edamame (in the pod)
- Sea salt to taste

Instructions:
1. Cook the edamame according to package instructions (usually by boiling or steaming).
2. Drain and sprinkle with sea salt.
3. Serve immediately for a protein-rich snack.

5. Apple and Peanut Butter Bites

Ingredients:
- 1 apple, cored and sliced into rounds
- 2 tablespoons powdered peanut butter (such as PB2), mixed with water to form a paste.

Instructions:
1. Wash and core the apple, then slice into rounds.

2. Spread a thin layer of the prepared powdered peanut butter on each apple slice.
3. Serve immediately for a sweet and satisfying snack.

These afternoon pick-me-ups are designed to keep you energized and focused throughout the day, helping you to stay on track with your healthy lifestyle. Enjoy these snacks as part of your journey to better health.

Dinner Delights: Delicious and Satisfying Zero-Point Dinner Ideas

Dinner is an important meal to conclude your day on a nutritious note. These zero-point dinner recipes are designed to be both delicious and satisfying, helping you stay on track with your weight loss goals. Here are five recipes, including Baked Lemon Herb Fish and Spaghetti Squash with Tomato Sauce:

1. Baked Lemon Herb Fish

Ingredients:
- 4 white fish fillets (such as cod or tilapia)
- 2 lemons, sliced
- 2 tablespoons fresh parsley, chopped
- 2 tablespoons fresh dill, chopped
- 2 garlic cloves, minced
- Salt and pepper to taste

Instructions:
1. Preheat the oven to 375°F (190°C).
2. Place the fish fillets on a baking sheet lined with parchment paper.
3. Sprinkle the minced garlic, parsley, dill, salt, and pepper evenly over the fish.
4. Arrange lemon slices on top of each fillet.
5. Bake for 15-20 minutes, or until the fish is cooked through and flakes easily with a fork.
6. Serve immediately with a side of steamed vegetables or a fresh salad.

2. Spaghetti Squash with Tomato Sauce

Ingredients:
- 1 large spaghetti squash
- 1 can (14.5 oz) diced tomatoes
- 1/2 cup onion, chopped
- 2 garlic cloves, minced
- 1 teaspoon olive oil (optional)
- 1 teaspoon dried oregano
- 1 teaspoon dried basil
- Salt and pepper to taste
- Fresh basil, for garnish

Instructions:
1. Preheat the oven to 400°F (200°C).
2. Cut the spaghetti squash in half lengthwise and remove the seeds.
3. Place the squash halves cut-side down on a baking sheet lined with parchment paper.
4. Bake for 40-45 minutes, or until the squash is tender.
5. While the squash is baking, heat olive oil in a pan over medium heat (if using).

6. Add the onion and garlic, and sauté until fragrant.
7. Add the diced tomatoes, oregano, basil, salt, and pepper.
8. Simmer the sauce for 10-15 minutes.
9. Once the squash is done, use a fork to scrape out the strands of spaghetti squash.
10. Serve the spaghetti squash topped with the tomato sauce and garnish with fresh basil.

3. Turkey and Vegetable Stir-Fry

Ingredients:
- 1 pound ground turkey breast
- 1 red bell pepper, sliced
- 1 yellow bell pepper, sliced
- 1 zucchini, sliced
- 1 cup snap peas
- 1 cup broccoli florets
- 2 garlic cloves, minced
- 1 tablespoon soy sauce (low sodium)
- 1 tablespoon rice vinegar
- 1 teaspoon ground ginger
- Fresh cilantro, for garnish

Instructions:

1. In a large skillet or wok, cook the ground turkey over medium heat until no longer pink. Remove from the skillet and set aside.
2. In the same skillet, add the bell peppers, zucchini, snap peas, broccoli, and garlic.
3. Stir-fry the vegetables for about 5-7 minutes until they are tender-crisp.
4. Return the turkey to the skillet.
5. Add soy sauce, rice vinegar, and ground ginger.
6. Stir well and cook for an additional 2-3 minutes to combine flavors.
7. Garnish with fresh cilantro and serve immediately.

4. Cauliflower Fried Rice

Ingredients:
- 1 medium head of cauliflower, grated or pulsed in a food processor to resemble rice
- 1 cup frozen peas and carrots, thawed
- 1/2 cup onion, chopped

- 2 garlic cloves, minced
- 2 large eggs, beaten
- 2 tablespoons soy sauce (low sodium)
- 1 teaspoon sesame oil (optional)
- Green onions, for garnish

Instructions:

1. In a large skillet or wok, heat sesame oil over medium heat (if using).
2. Add the onions and garlic, and sauté until fragrant.
3. Add the peas and carrots, and cook for about 2 minutes.
4. Push the vegetables to one side of the skillet and pour the beaten eggs into the other side.
5. Scramble the eggs until fully cooked.
6. Add the grated cauliflower and soy sauce to the skillet.
7. Stir-fry everything together for about 5-7 minutes, or until the cauliflower is tender.
8. Garnish with green onions and serve immediately.

5. Zucchini Noodles with Pesto

Ingredients:
- 4 medium zucchinis, spiralized into noodles
- 1 cup fresh basil leaves
- 1/4 cup pine nuts
- 2 garlic cloves
- 1/4 cup grated Parmesan cheese (optional)
- 1/4 cup olive oil (optional)
- Salt and pepper to taste
- Cherry tomatoes, halved (for garnish)

Instructions:
1. In a food processor, combine basil leaves, pine nuts, garlic, Parmesan cheese (if using), salt, and pepper.
2. Pulse until finely chopped.
3. With the processor running, slowly add olive oil through the feed tube until the pesto reaches your desired consistency.
4. In a large skillet, lightly sauté the zucchini noodles for 2-3 minutes until just tender.

5. Toss the zucchini noodles with the pesto sauce.

6. Garnish with cherry tomatoes and serve immediately.

These dinner delights are designed to be both filling and light, helping you enjoy your meals while staying committed to your healthy lifestyle. Enjoy these delicious recipes as part of your journey to better health.

Sweet Treats: Indulgent Yet Guilt-Free Desserts

Dessert doesn't have to derail your healthy eating plan. These zero-point sweet treats are indulgent yet guilt-free, allowing you to satisfy your sweet tooth while staying on track with your weight loss goals. Here are five delicious dessert recipes, including Frozen Fruit Sorbets and Baked Cinnamon Apples:

1. Frozen Fruit Sorbets

Ingredients:
- 2 cups frozen mixed berries (strawberries, blueberries, raspberries)
- 1 ripe banana, sliced and frozen
- Juice of 1 lemon
- 1 tablespoon honey or maple syrup (optional)

Instructions:
1. In a food processor or blender, combine the frozen mixed berries, frozen banana, and lemon juice.
2. Blend until smooth, stopping to scrape down the sides as needed.
3. Taste and add honey or maple syrup if desired for extra sweetness.
4. Serve immediately for a soft-serve consistency or transfer to a container and freeze for 1-2 hours for a firmer sorbet.
5. Scoop into bowls and enjoy.

2. Baked Cinnamon Apples

Ingredients:
- 4 large apples (such as Fuji or Honeycrisp), cored and sliced
- 1 teaspoon ground cinnamon
- 1/4 teaspoon ground nutmeg
- 1 tablespoon lemon juice
- 1/2 cup water

Instructions:
1. Preheat the oven to 375°F (190°C).
2. In a large bowl, toss the apple slices with cinnamon, nutmeg, and lemon juice.
3. Arrange the apple slices in a baking dish and pour water over them.
4. Cover the dish with foil and bake for 20-25 minutes, or until the apples are tender.
5. Serve warm, optionally with a dollop of non-fat Greek yogurt or a sprinkle of granola.

3. Chocolate Banana Nice Cream

Ingredients:
- 3 ripe bananas, sliced and frozen
- 2 tablespoons unsweetened cocoa powder
- 1 teaspoon vanilla extract
- 2 tablespoons almond milk (optional)

Instructions:
1. In a food processor or blender, combine the frozen banana slices, cocoa powder, and vanilla extract.
2. Blend until smooth, adding almond milk if needed for a creamier consistency.
3. Serve immediately for a soft-serve consistency or transfer to a container and freeze for 1-2 hours for a firmer nice cream.
4. Scoop into bowls and enjoy.

4. Berry Chia Pudding

Ingredients:
- 1 cup unsweetened almond milk
- 1/4 cup chia seeds

- 1 tablespoon honey or maple syrup (optional)
- 1/2 teaspoon vanilla extract
- 1 cup mixed berries (strawberries, blueberries, raspberries)

Instructions:

1. In a bowl, whisk together almond milk, chia seeds, honey or maple syrup (if using), and vanilla extract.
2. Let the mixture sit for 5 minutes, then whisk again to prevent clumping.
3. Cover and refrigerate for at least 2 hours or overnight until the chia seeds have absorbed the liquid and the mixture has thickened.
4. Stir well and divide the pudding into serving bowls.
5. Top with mixed berries and serve.

5. Mango Coconut Delight

Ingredients:

- 2 ripe mangoes, peeled and diced
- 1/2 cup unsweetened coconut milk

- 1 tablespoon lime juice
- 1 tablespoon honey or maple syrup (optional)
- 1/4 cup shredded coconut for garnish

Instructions:

1. In a blender, combine the diced mangoes, coconut milk, lime juice, and honey or maple syrup (if using).
2. Blend until smooth.
3. Pour the mixture into serving bowls or glasses.
4. Chill in the refrigerator for at least 1 hour before serving.
5. Garnish with shredded coconut and enjoy.

These indulgent yet guilt-free desserts will satisfy your cravings while keeping you on track with your healthy lifestyle. Enjoy these sweet treats as part of your journey to better health.

Hydration Heroes: Zero-Point Drinks and Smoothies to Stay Hydrated

Staying hydrated is essential for overall health and can also aid in weight loss. These zero-point drinks and smoothies are refreshing and hydrating, perfect for keeping you energized throughout the day. Here are five recipes, including Cucumber Mint Water and Green Detox Smoothie:

1. Cucumber Mint Water

Ingredients:
- 1/2 cucumber, thinly sliced
- 1/4 cup fresh mint leaves
- Ice cubes
- Water

Instructions:
1. In a large pitcher, combine cucumber slices and fresh mint leaves.
2. Fill the pitcher with ice cubes.
3. Add water to fill the pitcher.

4. Stir well and let it sit in the refrigerator for at least 1 hour to allow the flavors to infuse.
5. Serve chilled over ice.

2. Green Detox Smoothie

Ingredients:
- 1 cup spinach leaves
- 1/2 cup cucumber, chopped
- 1/2 cup celery, chopped
- 1/2 cup fresh parsley
- 1/2 green apple, chopped
- Juice of 1 lemon
- 1/2 cup water or coconut water
- Ice cubes (optional)

Instructions:
1. In a blender, combine spinach leaves, cucumber, celery, parsley, green apple, lemon juice, and water (or coconut water).
2. Blend until smooth and creamy.
3. Add ice cubes if desired for a colder smoothie.
4. Pour into glasses and serve immediately.

3. Berry Blast Smoothie

Ingredients:
- 1 cup mixed berries (strawberries, blueberries, raspberries)
- 1/2 banana, sliced and frozen
- 1 cup unsweetened almond milk or skim milk
- 1 tablespoon chia seeds (optional)
- Ice cubes

Instructions:
1. In a blender, combine mixed berries, frozen banana slices, almond milk (or skim milk), and chia seeds (if using).
2. Blend until smooth.
3. Add ice cubes for a thicker consistency, if desired.
4. Pour into glasses and serve immediately.

4. Citrus Infused Water
Ingredients:
- 1 orange, thinly sliced
- 1 lemon, thinly sliced
- 1 lime, thinly sliced

- Ice cubes
- Water

Instructions:
1. In a large pitcher, combine orange slices, lemon slices, and lime slices.
2. Fill the pitcher with ice cubes.
3. Add water to fill the pitcher.
4. Stir well and let it sit in the refrigerator for at least 1 hour to infuse the flavors.
5. Serve chilled over ice.

5. Tropical Coconut Water Smoothie

Ingredients:
- 1/2 cup coconut water
- 1/2 cup pineapple chunks
- 1/2 cup mango chunks
- 1/2 banana, sliced and frozen
- 1 tablespoon shredded coconut
- Ice cubes (optional)

Instructions:

1. In a blender, combine coconut water, pineapple chunks, mango chunks, frozen banana slices, and shredded coconut.
2. Blend until smooth and creamy.
3. Add ice cubes for a colder smoothie, if desired.
4. Pour into glasses and serve immediately.

These zero-point drinks and smoothies are not only hydrating but also packed with vitamins and minerals, making them perfect additions to your healthy lifestyle. Enjoy these refreshing beverages throughout the day to stay hydrated and energized.

Party Pleasers: Zero-Point Appetizers and Party Snacks

Hosting a gathering or attending a party doesn't have to mean sacrificing your healthy eating goals. These zero-point appetizers and party snacks are not only delicious but also guilt-free, allowing you to enjoy social occasions without the worry. Here are ten recipes, including Shrimp Cocktail and Stuffed Mushrooms:

1. Shrimp Cocktail

Ingredients:
- 1 pound cooked shrimp, peeled and deveined
- 1/2 cup ketchup
- 1/4 cup horseradish
- 1 tablespoon lemon juice
- 1 teaspoon Worcestershire sauce
- 1/2 teaspoon hot sauce (optional)
- Fresh parsley, for garnish
- Lemon wedges, for serving

Instructions:
1. In a bowl, combine ketchup, horseradish, lemon juice, Worcestershire sauce, and hot sauce (if using).
2. Mix well to combine.
3. Chill the sauce in the refrigerator for at least 30 minutes to allow the flavors to meld.
4. Arrange the cooked shrimp on a platter.

5. Serve the shrimp with the chilled cocktail sauce.

6. Garnish with fresh parsley and lemon wedges.

2. Stuffed Mushrooms

Ingredients:
- 12 large mushrooms, cleaned and stems removed
- 1/2 cup plain non-fat Greek yogurt
- 1/4 cup grated Parmesan cheese
- 1/4 cup chopped green onions
- 2 garlic cloves, minced
- 1/4 teaspoon dried thyme
- Salt and pepper to taste
- Fresh parsley, for garnish

Instructions:

1. Preheat the oven to 375°F (190°C).

2. In a bowl, mix together Greek yogurt, Parmesan cheese, green onions, minced garlic, dried thyme, salt, and pepper.

3. Spoon the mixture evenly into the mushroom caps.

4. Place the stuffed mushrooms on a baking sheet lined with parchment paper.
5. Bake for 20-25 minutes, or until the mushrooms are tender and the filling is golden brown.
6. Garnish with fresh parsley before serving.

3. Caprese Skewers

***Ingredients*:**
- Cherry tomatoes
- Fresh mozzarella balls
- Fresh basil leaves
- Balsamic glaze (optional)
- Wooden skewers

Instructions:

1. Thread a cherry tomato, a mozzarella ball, and a basil leaf onto each skewer.
2. Arrange the skewers on a serving platter.
3. Drizzle with balsamic glaze, if desired, before serving.

4. Cucumber Cups with Tuna Salad

Ingredients:
- 2 cucumbers, cut into thick slices
- 1 can (5 oz) tuna, drained
- 1/4 cup plain non-fat Greek yogurt
- 1 tablespoon Dijon mustard
- 1 tablespoon fresh dill, chopped
- Salt and pepper to taste

Instructions:
1. Scoop out the centers of the cucumber slices to create cups.
2. In a bowl, mix together tuna, Greek yogurt, Dijon mustard, chopped dill, salt, and pepper.
3. Spoon the tuna salad into the cucumber cups.
4. Arrange on a serving platter and serve chilled.

5. Grilled Vegetable Skewers

Ingredients:
- Assorted vegetables (such as bell peppers, zucchini, cherry tomatoes, mushrooms)
- Wooden skewers

- 1 tablespoon olive oil
- 1 teaspoon Italian seasoning
- Salt and pepper to taste

Instructions:

1. Preheat the grill or grill pan over medium-high heat.
2. Cut the vegetables into bite-sized pieces.
3. Thread the vegetables onto skewers, alternating colors and varieties.
4. In a small bowl, mix olive oil, Italian seasoning, salt, and pepper.
5. Brush the vegetable skewers with the olive oil mixture.
6. Grill for 8-10 minutes, turning occasionally, until the vegetables are tender and slightly charred.
7. Serve immediately.

6. Deviled Eggs

Ingredients:

- 6 hard-boiled eggs, peeled and halved
- 2 tablespoons plain non-fat Greek yogurt

- 1 tablespoon Dijon mustard
- 1 tablespoon chopped chives
- Paprika for garnish
- Salt and pepper to taste

Instructions:
1. Carefully remove the yolks from the egg halves and place them in a bowl.
2. Mash the egg yolks with Greek yogurt, Dijon mustard, chopped chives, salt, and pepper until smooth.
3. Spoon or pipe the yolk mixture back into the egg white halves.
4. Sprinkle with paprika for garnish.
5. Serve chilled.

7. Antipasto Skewers

Ingredients:
- Slices of low-sodium deli turkey or ham
- Cherry tomatoes
- Mozzarella cheese cubes
- Olives (black or green)
- Basil leaves

- Balsamic glaze (optional)
- Wooden skewers

Instructions:
1. Thread a slice of deli meat, a cherry tomato, a mozzarella cube, an olive, and a basil leaf onto each skewer.
2. Arrange the skewers on a serving platter.
3. Drizzle with balsamic glaze, if desired, before serving.

8. Zucchini Roll-Ups

Ingredients:
- 1 large zucchini, thinly sliced lengthwise
- 1/2 cup plain non-fat Greek yogurt
- 1/4 cup grated Parmesan cheese
- 1/4 cup sun-dried tomatoes, chopped
- Fresh basil leaves
- Salt and pepper to taste.

Instructions:
1. Lay the zucchini slices flat on a cutting board or plate.

2. In a bowl, mix together Greek yogurt, Parmesan cheese, chopped sun-dried tomatoes, salt, and pepper.
3. Spread a thin layer of the yogurt mixture onto each zucchini slice.
4. Place a basil leaf on one end of each zucchini slice and roll up tightly.
5. Secure with a toothpick if needed and arrange on a serving platter.

9. Gazpacho Shooters

Ingredients:
- 2 cups diced tomatoes
- 1 cucumber, peeled and diced
- 1/2 red bell pepper, diced
- 1/4 cup red onion, diced
- 1 garlic clove, minced
- 2 tablespoons olive oil
- 2 tablespoons red wine vinegar
- 1/2 teaspoon cumin
- Salt and pepper to taste
- Fresh cilantro for garnish

Instructions:
1. In a blender or food processor, combine diced tomatoes, cucumber, red bell pepper, red onion, minced garlic, olive oil, red wine vinegar, cumin, salt, and pepper.
2. Blend until smooth.
3. Chill the gazpacho in the refrigerator for at least 1 hour before serving.
4. Pour the gazpacho into shot glasses or small cups.
5. Garnish with fresh cilantro before serving.

10. Smoked Salmon Cucumber Bites

Ingredients:
- 1 English cucumber, sliced into rounds
- 4 oz smoked salmon, cut into small pieces
- 1/4 cup plain non-fat Greek yogurt
- -1 tablespoon fresh dill, chopped
- Lemon zest for garnish

Instructions:
1. Arrange the cucumber rounds on a serving platter.

2. In a bowl, mix together Greek yogurt and chopped dill.
3. Spoon a small dollop of the yogurt mixture onto each cucumber round.
4. Top with a piece of smoked salmon.
5. Garnish with lemon zest before serving.

These zero-point appetizers and party snacks are sure to be a hit at any gathering, allowing you to enjoy delicious flavors while maintaining your healthy lifestyle. Enjoy these recipes with friends and family as part of your journey to better health.

On-the-Go Options: Portable Zero-Point Snacks and Meals

When you're on-the-go, having nutritious and satisfying zero-point snacks and meals ready can keep you on track with your health goals. These recipes are perfect for packing and enjoying wherever your day takes you, including Mason Jar Salads and Protein-Packed Snack Bars:

Mason Jar Salads

Ingredients:
- 1 pint-size mason jar with lid
- 2 tablespoons balsamic vinaigrette dressing (or dressing of choice)
- 1/4 cup cherry tomatoes, halved
- 1/4 cup cucumber, diced
- 1/4 cup bell pepper, diced
- 1/4 cup shredded carrots
- 1/4 cup red cabbage, shredded
- 1/4 cup chickpeas, rinsed and drained
- 1 cup mixed salad greens

Instructions:
1. Pour the dressing into the bottom of the mason jar.
2. Layer cherry tomatoes, cucumber, bell pepper, shredded carrots, red cabbage, and chickpeas in the jar.

3. Top with mixed salad greens, packing them down lightly.

4. Seal the mason jar tightly with the lid and refrigerate until ready to eat.

5. When ready to eat, shake the jar to distribute the dressing evenly.

6. Pour the salad into a bowl and enjoy.

Protein-Packed Snack Bars

Ingredients:
- 1 cup old-fashioned oats
- 1/2 cup unsweetened applesauce
- 1/4 cup honey or maple syrup
- 1/4 cup almond butter or peanut butter
- 1/2 cup protein powder (vanilla or chocolate)
- 1/4 cup unsweetened almond milk or skim milk
- 1/2 cup dried cranberries or raisins
- 1/4 cup chopped nuts (almonds, walnuts, or pecans)
- 1/4 cup dark chocolate chips (optional)

Instructions:
1. Preheat the oven to 350°F (175°C). Line an 8x8-inch baking dish with parchment paper.
2. In a large bowl, combine oats, applesauce, honey (or maple syrup), almond butter (or peanut butter), protein powder, and almond milk (or skim milk). Mix until well combined.
3. Fold in dried cranberries (or raisins), chopped nuts, and dark chocolate chips (if using).
4. Press the mixture evenly into the prepared baking dish.
5. Bake for 15-20 minutes, or until the edges are golden brown.
6. Allow the bars to cool completely in the baking dish before cutting into squares or bars.
7. Store in an airtight container for up to one week.

Fruit and Yogurt Parfait

Ingredients:
- 1 cup plain non-fat Greek yogurt
- 1/2 cup mixed berries (strawberries, blueberries, raspberries)

- 1/4 cup granola (choose a zero-point granola or homemade)
- 1 tablespoon honey or maple syrup (optional)

Instructions:
1. In a glass or portable container, layer Greek yogurt, mixed berries, and granola.
2. Drizzle with honey or maple syrup, if desired.
3. Seal tightly and keep refrigerated until ready to eat.
4. Stir before eating to combine all the flavors.

Veggie and Hummus Snack Box

Ingredients:
- Baby carrots
- Cucumber slices
- Cherry tomatoes
- Sugar snap peas
- Radish slices
- 1/4 cup hummus (store-bought or homemade)

Instructions:
1. Arrange baby carrots, cucumber slices, cherry tomatoes, sugar snap peas, and radish slices in a portable container or bento box.
2. Pack hummus in a separate small container or compartment.
3. Seal the containers tightly and keep refrigerated until ready to eat.
4. Dip veggies in hummus for a satisfying and nutritious snack.

Tuna Lettuce Wraps

Ingredients:
- 1 can (5 oz) tuna, drained
- 1 tablespoon plain non-fat Greek yogurt
- 1 teaspoon Dijon mustard
- 1/4 cup diced celery
- 1/4 cup diced red onion
- Salt and pepper to taste
- Butter lettuce leaves

Instructions:
1. In a bowl, mix together tuna, Greek yogurt, Dijon mustard, diced celery, and diced red onion.
2. Season with salt and pepper to taste.
3. Spoon tuna mixture onto butter lettuce leaves.
4. Roll up the lettuce leaves and secure with toothpicks if needed.
5. Pack in a portable container or wrap tightly in foil.
6. Keep refrigerated until ready to eat.

Turkey and Cheese Roll-Ups

Ingredients:
- 4 slices low-sodium deli turkey
- 4 slices reduced-fat cheese (such as cheddar or Swiss)
- 1/4 cup baby spinach leaves
- Mustard or hummus for spreading (optional)

Instructions:
1. Lay out turkey slices on a clean surface.

2. Spread each slice with mustard or hummus, if using.

3. Place a slice of cheese on top of each turkey slice.

4. Arrange baby spinach leaves on top of the cheese.

5. Roll up tightly and secure with toothpicks if needed.

6. Pack in a portable container or wrap tightly in foil.

7. Keep refrigerated until ready to eat.

Greek Yogurt and Berry Smoothie

Ingredients:
- 1 cup plain non-fat Greek yogurt
- 1/2 cup mixed berries (strawberries, blueberries, raspberries)
- 1/2 banana, sliced and frozen
- 1/2 cup unsweetened almond milk or skim milk
- 1 tablespoon chia seeds (optional)
- Ice cubes (optional)

Instructions:

1. In a blender, combine Greek yogurt, mixed berries, frozen banana slices, almond milk (or skim milk), and chia seeds (if using).
2. Blend until smooth and creamy.
3. Add ice cubes for a thicker consistency, if desired.
4. Pour into a portable container or insulated tumbler.
5. Keep chilled until ready to drink.

Quinoa Salad Jars

Ingredients:
- 1 cup cooked quinoa
- 1/2 cup cherry tomatoes, halved
- 1/2 cup cucumber, diced
- 1/4 cup red onion, finely chopped
- 1/4 cup Kalamata olives, chopped
- 1/4 cup crumbled feta cheese
- 2 tablespoons olive oil
- 1 tablespoon red wine vinegar
- Salt and pepper to taste

***Instructions*:**
1. In each mason jar, layer cooked quinoa, cherry tomatoes, cucumber, red onion, Kalamata olives, and crumbled feta cheese.
2. In a small bowl, whisk together olive oil, red wine vinegar, salt, and pepper.
3. Pour the dressing over the salad in each jar.
4. Seal tightly with lids and refrigerate until ready to eat.
5. Shake the jar before eating to distribute the dressing.

Egg Muffins

***Ingredients*:**
- 6 eggs
- 1/4 cup unsweetened almond milk or skim milk
- 1/2 cup diced bell peppers
- 1/2 cup diced spinach
- 1/4 cup diced onion
- Salt and pepper to taste

Instructions:
1. Preheat the oven to 350°F (175°C). Grease a muffin tin with cooking spray.
2. In a bowl, whisk together eggs, almond milk (or skim milk), diced bell peppers, diced spinach, diced onion, salt, and pepper.
3. Pour the egg mixture evenly into the muffin tin, filling each cup about 3/4 full.
4. Bake for 20-25 minutes, or until the egg muffins are set and lightly golden.
5. Allow to cool slightly before removing from the muffin tin.
6. Store in an airtight container in the refrigerator.
7. Reheat in the microwave for a quick and portable breakfast or snack.

Cauliflower Fried Rice

Ingredients:
- 1 head cauliflower, grated or finely chopped
- 1 cup mixed vegetables (peas, carrots, corn)

- 1/2 cup diced bell peppers
- 1/4 cup diced onion
- 2 cloves garlic, minced
- 2 tablespoons low-sodium soy sauce
- 1 tablespoon sesame oil
- 2 eggs, beaten (optional)
- Salt and pepper to taste

Instructions:

1. In a large skillet or wok, heat sesame oil over medium heat.
2. Add diced bell peppers, diced onion, and minced garlic. Sauté for 3-5 minutes until vegetables are tender.
3. Stir in grated cauliflower and mixed vegetables. Cook for another 5 minutes, stirring occasionally.
4. Push the cauliflower mixture to one side of the skillet.
5. Pour beaten eggs into the empty side of the skillet and scramble until cooked through.
6. Stir everything together in the skillet.
7. Season with low-sodium soy sauce, salt, and pepper to taste.

8. Allow to cool slightly before portioning into portable containers.

9. Store in the refrigerator and reheat in the microwave before serving.

These portable zero-point snacks and meals are perfect for busy days, ensuring you have nutritious options at your fingertips wherever you go. Prepare them ahead of time and enjoy the convenience of healthy eating on-the-go.

Kid-Friendly Favorites: Zero-Point Recipes

Creating kid-friendly zero-point recipes can be both fun and nutritious. Here are some recipes including Mini Veggie Pizzas and Banana Ice Cream that kids will enjoy:

1. Mini Veggie Pizzas

Ingredients:
- Whole wheat English muffins

- 1/2 cup tomato sauce (choose a sugar-free option)
- 1/2 cup shredded mozzarella cheese (reduced-fat)
- Assorted veggies (bell peppers, cherry tomatoes, mushrooms, spinach)
- Italian seasoning

Instructions:
1. Preheat the oven to 375°F (190°C).
2. Split the English muffins in half and place them on a baking sheet.
3. Spread tomato sauce evenly on each muffin half.
4. Sprinkle shredded mozzarella cheese over the sauce.
5. Top with assorted veggies and sprinkle with Italian seasoning.
6. Bake for 10-12 minutes, or until the cheese is melted and bubbly.
7. Allow to cool slightly before serving.

2. Banana Ice Cream

Ingredients:
- 4 ripe bananas, peeled and sliced
- 1/2 teaspoon vanilla extract
- Optional mix-ins: chocolate chips, strawberries, nuts

Instructions:
1. Place sliced bananas on a baking sheet lined with parchment paper.
2. Freeze bananas for at least 2 hours, or until firm.
3. Transfer frozen bananas to a food processor.
4. Add vanilla extract.
5. Blend until smooth and creamy, scraping down the sides as needed.
6. Add optional mix-ins if desired and pulse to combine.
7. Serve immediately as soft-serve or freeze for 1-2 hours for a firmer texture.

3. Veggie Quesadillas

__Ingredients__:
- Whole wheat tortillas
- 1/2 cup black beans, drained and rinsed
- 1/2 cup shredded cheddar cheese (reduced-fat)
- Assorted veggies (bell peppers, corn, spinach)
- Salsa and Greek yogurt (optional, for dipping)

__Instructions__:
1. Heat a large skillet over medium heat.
2. Place one tortilla in the skillet and sprinkle with half of the shredded cheese.
3. Add black beans, assorted veggies, and remaining cheese.
4. Top with another tortilla and press down gently.
5. Cook for 3-4 minutes on each side, or until tortilla is golden brown and cheese is melted.
6. Remove from skillet and let cool slightly before slicing into wedges.

7. Serve with salsa and Greek yogurt for dipping.

4. Apple Sandwiches

Ingredients:
- 1 apple, cored and sliced into rounds
- Peanut butter (sugar-free)
- Granola (choose a zero-point option or homemade)

Instructions:
1. Spread peanut butter on one side of apple slices.
2. Sprinkle granola over the peanut butter.
3. Top with another apple slice to form a sandwich.
4. Repeat with remaining apple slices.
5. Serve immediately or wrap tightly and refrigerate until ready to eat.

5. Veggie Nuggets

Ingredients:
- 1 cup cooked quinoa
- 1 cup mashed sweet potatoes
- 1/2 cup finely chopped mixed veggies (carrots, peas, corn)
- 1/2 cup grated cheese (reduced-fat)
- 1/4 cup whole wheat breadcrumbs
- 1 egg, beaten
- Salt and pepper to taste
- Cooking spray

Instructions:
1. Preheat the oven to 400°F (200°C). Line a baking sheet with parchment paper and spray with cooking spray.
2. In a large bowl, combine cooked quinoa, mashed sweet potatoes, chopped veggies, grated cheese, breadcrumbs, egg, salt, and pepper.
3. Mix until well combined.
4. Shape mixture into small nuggets and place on the prepared baking sheet.

5. Bake for 20-25 minutes, flipping halfway through, until nuggets are golden and crispy.
6. Allow to cool slightly before serving with dipping sauce of choice.

6. Berry Smoothie Popsicles

Ingredients:
- 1 cup mixed berries (strawberries, blueberries, raspberries)
- 1 cup plain non-fat Greek yogurt
- 1 tablespoon honey or maple syrup (optional)

Instructions:
1. In a blender, combine mixed berries, Greek yogurt, and honey (or maple syrup, if using).
2. Blend until smooth and creamy.
3. Pour mixture into popsicle molds.
4. Insert popsicle sticks and freeze for at least 4 hours, or until firm.
5. Remove from molds and serve immediately.

7. Zucchini Tots
Ingredients:
- 2 cups grated zucchini
- 1/2 cup shredded cheese (reduced-fat)
- 1/4 cup whole wheat breadcrumbs
- 1 egg, beaten
- Salt and pepper to taste
- Cooking spray

Instructions:
1. Preheat the oven to 400°F (200°C). Line a baking sheet with parchment paper and spray with cooking spray.
2. Place grated zucchini in a clean kitchen towel and squeeze out excess moisture.
3. In a bowl, combine squeezed zucchini, shredded cheese, breadcrumbs, egg, salt, and pepper.
4. Mix until well combined.
5. Shape mixture into small tots and place on the prepared baking sheet.
6. Bake for 15-20 minutes, flipping halfway through, until tots are golden and crispy.

7. Allow to cool slightly before serving with ketchup or ranch dressing for dipping.

8. Cucumber Sushi Rolls

Ingredients:
- 1 cucumber
- 1/2 cup cooked quinoa
- 1/4 cup shredded carrots
- 1/4 cup avocado, sliced
- 1/4 cup cucumber, julienned
- Soy sauce or tamari (low-sodium, for dipping)

Instructions:
1. Peel cucumber into thin strips using a vegetable peeler, leaving skin on for color.
2. Lay cucumber strips flat and spread a thin layer of quinoa over each strip.
3. Add shredded carrots, avocado slices, and julienned cucumber on top of quinoa.
4. Roll cucumber strips tightly into sushi rolls.
5. Slice rolls into bite-sized pieces and serve with soy sauce or tamari for dipping.

9. Sweet Potato Fries

Ingredients:
- 2 medium sweet potatoes, peeled and cut into thin strips
- 1 tablespoon olive oil
- 1/2 teaspoon paprika
- 1/2 teaspoon garlic powder
- Salt and pepper to taste

Instructions:
1. Preheat the oven to 425°F (220°C). Line a baking sheet with parchment paper.
2. In a large bowl, toss sweet potato strips with olive oil, paprika, garlic powder, salt, and pepper.
3. Arrange sweet potato strips in a single layer on the prepared baking sheet.
4. Bake for 20-25 minutes, flipping halfway through, until fries are golden and crispy.
5. Allow to cool slightly before serving with ketchup or Greek yogurt for dipping.

10. Watermelon Pops

Ingredients:
- Watermelon slices, cut into triangles or sticks
- Wooden popsicle sticks

Instructions:
1. Insert a popsicle stick into the rind of each watermelon slice.
2. Place watermelon pops on a baking sheet lined with parchment paper.
3. Freeze for at least 2 hours, or until firm.
4. Serve immediately as a refreshing and hydrating treat.

These kid-friendly zero-point recipes are not only nutritious but also delicious, making them perfect for children of all ages. Enjoy creating these wholesome dishes together and promoting healthy eating habits in a fun and enjoyable way!

Cultural Cuisine: Zero-Point Recipes Inspired by Global Flavors

Creating zero-point recipes inspired by global flavors adds variety and excitement to your meals. Here are some recipes including Mexican Cauliflower Rice and Thai Cucumber Salad:

1. Mexican Cauliflower Rice

Ingredients:
- 1 medium head cauliflower, grated or finely chopped
- 1 tablespoon olive oil
- 1/2 cup diced onion
- 1/2 cup diced bell peppers (red, yellow, or green)
- 1 jalapeño, seeded and minced (optional)
- 1 teaspoon ground cumin
- 1/2 teaspoon chili powder
- Salt and pepper to taste
- Fresh cilantro, chopped (for garnish)

Instructions:

1. Heat olive oil in a large skillet over medium heat.
2. Add diced onion, bell peppers, and jalapeño (if using). Sauté until vegetables are tender, about 5 minutes.
3. Stir in ground cumin and chili powder, cooking for an additional minute until fragrant.
4. Add grated cauliflower to the skillet, stirring to combine with the seasoned vegetables.
5. Cook for 5-7 minutes, or until cauliflower is tender but still slightly crisp.
6. Season with salt and pepper to taste.
7. Garnish with fresh chopped cilantro before serving.

2. Thai Cucumber Salad

Ingredients:
- 2 cucumbers, thinly sliced
- 1/4 cup red onion, thinly sliced
- 1/4 cup fresh cilantro, chopped
- 1/4 cup fresh mint leaves, chopped
- 1/4 cup rice vinegar

- 1 tablespoon soy sauce (low-sodium)
- 1 tablespoon lime juice
- 1 tablespoon honey or agave syrup
- 1 teaspoon sesame oil
- Red pepper flakes (optional, for heat)
- Salt and pepper to taste

Instructions:

1. In a large bowl, combine sliced cucumbers, red onion, cilantro, and mint leaves.
2. In a small bowl, whisk together rice vinegar, soy sauce, lime juice, honey (or agave syrup), sesame oil, and red pepper flakes (if using).
3. Pour dressing over cucumber mixture, tossing gently to coat.
4. Season with salt and pepper to taste.
5. Let marinate in the refrigerator for at least 30 minutes before serving to allow flavors to meld.
6. Serve chilled as a refreshing side dish or light salad.

3. Greek Chickpea Salad

Ingredients:

- 1 can (15 oz) chickpeas, rinsed and drained
- 1 cucumber, diced
- 1/2 cup cherry tomatoes, halved
- 1/4 cup red onion, finely chopped
- 1/4 cup Kalamata olives, sliced
- 1/4 cup crumbled feta cheese
- 2 tablespoons olive oil
- 1 tablespoon red wine vinegar
- 1 teaspoon dried oregano
- Salt and pepper to taste

Instructions:

1. In a large bowl, combine chickpeas, diced cucumber, cherry tomatoes, red onion, Kalamata olives, and crumbled feta cheese.
2. In a small bowl, whisk together olive oil, red wine vinegar, dried oregano, salt, and pepper.
3. Pour dressing over salad ingredients, tossing gently to combine.

4. Let sit at room temperature for 10-15 minutes to allow flavors to meld before serving.
5. Serve as a light and satisfying salad or side dish.

4. Japanese Miso Soup

Ingredients:
- 4 cups water
- 2 tablespoons miso paste
- 1 block tofu, cubed
- 1 cup seaweed (such as wakame), rehydrated if dried
- 1 green onion, thinly sliced
- Optional: sliced mushrooms, grated ginger

Instructions:
1. In a medium pot, bring water to a boil.
2. Reduce heat to low and whisk in miso paste until dissolved.
3. Add tofu cubes and seaweed to the pot.
4. Simmer for 5-7 minutes, stirring occasionally, until tofu is heated through and seaweed is tender.

5. Remove from heat and stir in sliced green onions.

6. Serve hot as a comforting and nourishing soup.

5. Indian Chickpea Curry (Chana Masala)

Ingredients:
- 1 can (15 oz) chickpeas, rinsed and drained
- 1 onion, finely chopped
- 2 cloves garlic, minced
- 1 tablespoon grated ginger
- 1 can (15 oz) diced tomatoes
- 1/2 cup vegetable broth
- 1 teaspoon ground cumin
- 1 teaspoon ground coriander
- 1/2 teaspoon turmeric powder
- 1/2 teaspoon paprika
- 1/4 teaspoon cayenne pepper (adjust to taste)
- Salt and pepper to taste
- Fresh cilantro, chopped (for garnish)

Instructions:

1. Heat olive oil in a large skillet over medium heat.
2. Add chopped onion and sauté until translucent, about 5 minutes.
3. Stir in minced garlic and grated ginger, cooking for an additional minute until fragrant.
4. Add diced tomatoes (with juices) and vegetable broth to the skillet, stirring to combine.
5. Add ground cumin, ground coriander, turmeric powder, paprika, and cayenne pepper to the skillet, stirring to evenly distribute spices.
6. Bring mixture to a simmer and cook for 10 minutes, allowing flavors to meld and sauce to thicken.
7. Add chickpeas to the skillet, stirring to coat with the sauce.
8. Cook for an additional 5-7 minutes, or until chickpeas are heated through.
9. Season with salt and pepper to taste.
10. Garnish with fresh chopped cilantro before serving.

6. Italian Caprese Salad

Ingredients:
- 2 large tomatoes, sliced
- 1 ball fresh mozzarella cheese, sliced
- Fresh basil leaves
- Balsamic vinegar glaze
- Salt and pepper to taste

Instructions:
1. Arrange alternating slices of tomato and mozzarella cheese on a serving platter.
2. Tuck fresh basil leaves between tomato and cheese slices.
3. Drizzle balsamic vinegar glaze over the salad.
4. Season with salt and pepper to taste.
5. Serve immediately as a refreshing and elegant salad.

7. Korean Cucumber Kimchi

Ingredients:
- 2 cucumbers, thinly sliced
- 1 tablespoon coarse sea salt

- 1/4 cup Korean red pepper flakes (gochugaru)
- 2 cloves garlic, minced
- 1 tablespoon grated ginger
- 1 tablespoon soy sauce (low-sodium)
- 1 tablespoon rice vinegar
- 1 tablespoon honey or agave syrup
- 1 green onion, thinly sliced

Instructions:
1. Place cucumber slices in a large bowl and sprinkle with coarse sea salt.
2. Toss cucumbers to coat evenly with salt and let sit for 30 minutes.
3. Rinse cucumbers thoroughly under cold water to remove excess salt.
4. In a separate bowl, combine Korean red pepper flakes, minced garlic, grated ginger, soy sauce, rice vinegar, and honey (or agave syrup).
5. Add rinsed cucumber slices and green onion to the bowl, tossing gently to coat with the seasoning mixture.
6. Transfer cucumber kimchi to a clean jar or container with a tight-fitting lid.

7. Refrigerate for at least 2 hours, or overnight, to allow flavors to develop before serving.

8. Moroccan Spiced Lentil Soup

Ingredients:
- 1 cup dried lentils, rinsed and drained
- 1 onion, finely chopped
- 2 carrots, diced
- 2 celery stalks, diced
- 2 cloves garlic, minced
- 1 tablespoon olive oil
- 1 teaspoon ground cumin
- 1 teaspoon ground coriander
- 1/2 teaspoon ground turmeric
- 1/2 teaspoon ground cinnamon
- 4 cups vegetable broth
- 1 can (14 oz) diced tomatoes
- Salt and pepper to taste
- Fresh cilantro, chopped (for garnish)

Instructions:
1. In a large pot, heat olive oil over medium heat.

2. Add chopped onion, diced carrots, and diced celery to the pot. Sauté until vegetables are softened, about 5-7 minutes.

3. Stir in minced garlic, ground cumin, ground coriander, ground turmeric, and ground cinnamon, cooking for an additional minute until fragrant.

4. Add rinsed lentils, vegetable broth, and diced tomatoes (with juices) to the pot.

5. Bring soup to a boil, then reduce heat to low and simmer for 20-25 minutes, or until lentils are tender.

6. Season with salt and pepper to taste.

7. Garnish with fresh chopped cilantro before serving.

Comfort Food Classics: Zero-Point Versions

Creating zero-point versions of classic comfort foods can satisfy cravings while supporting a healthy lifestyle. Here are some recipes including Cauliflower Mac and Cheese and Turkey Chili:

1. Cauliflower Mac and Cheese

Ingredients:
- 1 medium head cauliflower, cut into florets
- 1 cup fat-free Greek yogurt
- 1 cup fat-free cottage cheese
- 1 cup shredded reduced-fat cheddar cheese
- 1/2 teaspoon garlic powder
- Salt and pepper to taste
- Chopped fresh parsley (for garnish)

Instructions:
1. Preheat oven to 375°F (190°C). Grease a baking dish with cooking spray.
2. Steam cauliflower florets until tender, about 5-7 minutes. Drain well and set aside.
3. In a blender or food processor, combine Greek yogurt, cottage cheese, shredded cheddar cheese, garlic powder, salt, and pepper. Blend until smooth.

4. In a large bowl, mix together steamed cauliflower and cheese sauce until cauliflower is well coated.
5. Transfer mixture to the prepared baking dish and spread evenly.
6. Bake for 20-25 minutes, or until hot and bubbly.
7. Garnish with chopped parsley before serving.

2. Turkey Chili

Ingredients:
- 1 lb lean ground turkey
- 1 onion, chopped
- 3 cloves garlic, minced
- 1 bell pepper, diced
- 1 can (15 oz) kidney beans, rinsed and drained
- 1 can (15 oz) black beans, rinsed and drained
- 1 can (15 oz) diced tomatoes
- 1 cup low-sodium chicken broth
- 2 tablespoons tomato paste
- 1 tablespoon chili powder

- 1 teaspoon ground cumin
- 1/2 teaspoon paprika
- Salt and pepper to taste
- Chopped fresh cilantro (for garnish)
- Fat-free Greek yogurt (optional, for serving)

Instructions:

1. In a large pot or Dutch oven, cook ground turkey over medium heat until browned, breaking it up with a spoon as it cooks.
2. Add chopped onion, minced garlic, and diced bell pepper to the pot. Cook until vegetables are softened, about 5 minutes.
3. Stir in kidney beans, black beans, diced tomatoes (with juices), chicken broth, tomato paste, chili powder, ground cumin, paprika, salt, and pepper.
4. Bring chili to a boil, then reduce heat to low and simmer for 20-25 minutes, stirring occasionally.
5. Adjust seasoning with additional salt and pepper if needed.

6. Serve hot, garnished with chopped cilantro and a dollop of fat-free Greek yogurt if desired.

3. Spinach and Mushroom Lasagna

Ingredients:
- 9 whole wheat lasagna noodles, cooked according to package instructions
- 1 lb fresh spinach, washed and chopped
- 8 oz mushrooms, sliced
- 1 onion, chopped
- 3 cloves garlic, minced
- 1 can (15 oz) low-fat ricotta cheese
- 1 cup shredded part-skim mozzarella cheese
- 1/2 cup grated Parmesan cheese
- 1 jar (24 oz) marinara sauce (sugar-free)
- 1 tablespoon olive oil
- Salt and pepper to taste
- Fresh basil leaves (for garnish)

Instructions:
1. Preheat oven to 375°F (190°C). Grease a 9x13-inch baking dish with cooking spray.

2. In a large skillet, heat olive oil over medium heat. Add chopped onion and sliced mushrooms, cooking until softened, about 5-7 minutes.
3. Stir in minced garlic and chopped spinach, cooking until spinach is wilted.
4. In a bowl, combine ricotta cheese, shredded mozzarella cheese, and grated Parmesan cheese. Season with salt and pepper.
5. Spread 1/3 of marinara sauce evenly on the bottom of the prepared baking dish.
6. Layer with 3 cooked lasagna noodles, followed by half of the spinach-mushroom mixture and half of the cheese mixture.
7. Repeat layers: marinara sauce, lasagna noodles, remaining spinach-mushroom mixture, and remaining cheese mixture.
8. Top with remaining marinara sauce and sprinkle with additional shredded mozzarella cheese if desired.
9. Cover with foil and bake for 30 minutes.
10. Remove foil and bake for an additional 10 minutes, or until lasagna is bubbly and cheese is melted.

11. Let lasagna rest for 10 minutes before serving. Garnish with fresh basil leaves.

4. Chicken and Vegetable Stir-Fry

Ingredients:
- 1 lb boneless, skinless chicken breast, thinly sliced
- 2 cups broccoli florets
- 1 bell pepper, sliced
- 1 cup sliced carrots
- 1 cup snow peas
- 3 cloves garlic, minced
- 1 tablespoon grated ginger
- 1/4 cup low-sodium soy sauce
- 2 tablespoons hoisin sauce
- 1 tablespoon cornstarch
- 1 tablespoon olive oil
- Cooked brown rice (optional, for serving)
- Chopped green onions (for garnish)

Instructions:
1. In a small bowl, whisk together soy sauce, hoisin sauce, and cornstarch. Set aside.

2. Heat olive oil in a large skillet or wok over medium-high heat.
3. Add sliced chicken breast to the skillet, cooking until browned and cooked through, about 5-7 minutes.
4. Remove chicken from skillet and set aside.
5. Add broccoli florets, sliced bell pepper, sliced carrots, and snow peas to the skillet. Cook until vegetables are tender-crisp, about 5 minutes.
6. Stir in minced garlic and grated ginger, cooking for an additional minute until fragrant.
7. Return cooked chicken to the skillet.
8. Pour soy sauce mixture over chicken and vegetables, stirring to coat evenly. Cook for 2-3 minutes, or until sauce thickens.
9. Serve hot over cooked brown rice if desired, garnished with chopped green onions.

5. Butternut Squash Soup

Ingredients:

- 1 medium butternut squash, peeled, seeded, and diced
- 1 onion, chopped

- 2 carrots, chopped
- 2 celery stalks, chopped
- 4 cups low-sodium vegetable broth
- 1 teaspoon ground cinnamon
- 1/2 teaspoon ground nutmeg
- Salt and pepper to taste
- Fat-free Greek yogurt (for serving, optional)
- Fresh thyme leaves (for garnish)

Instructions:

1. In a large pot, combine diced butternut squash, chopped onion, chopped carrots, chopped celery, and vegetable broth.
2. Bring mixture to a boil, then reduce heat to low and simmer for 20-25 minutes, or until vegetables are tender.
3. Use an immersion blender to puree soup until smooth. Alternatively, carefully transfer soup in batches to a blender and blend until smooth, then return to the pot.
4. Stir in ground cinnamon and ground nutmeg. Season with salt and pepper to taste.

5. Serve hot, garnished with a dollop of fat-free Greek yogurt and fresh thyme leaves.

6. Stuffed Bell Peppers

Ingredients:
- 4 bell peppers, tops cut off and seeds removed
- 1 lb lean ground turkey or chicken
- 1 onion, chopped
- 2 cloves garlic, minced
- 1 cup cooked quinoa
- 1 can (15 oz) diced tomatoes, drained
- 1 cup shredded reduced-fat cheddar cheese
- 1 teaspoon dried oregano
- 1 teaspoon dried basil
- Salt and pepper to taste

Instructions:
1. Preheat oven to 375°F (190°C). Grease a baking dish with cooking spray.

2. In a large skillet, cook ground turkey or chicken over medium heat until browned, breaking it up with a spoon as it cooks.

3. Add chopped onion and minced garlic to the skillet. Cook until onion is translucent, about 5 minutes.

4. Stir in cooked quinoa, drained diced tomatoes, shredded cheddar cheese, dried oregano, dried basil, salt, and pepper.

5. Spoon turkey mixture evenly into hollowed-out bell peppers.

6. Place stuffed bell peppers upright in the prepared baking dish.

7. Cover dish with foil and bake for 30 minutes.

8. Remove foil and bake for an additional 10-15 minutes, or until bell peppers are tender and filling is heated through.

9. Serve hot, garnished with fresh herbs if desired.

7. Eggplant Parmesan

Ingredients:
- 1 large eggplant, thinly sliced
- 1 cup whole wheat breadcrumbs
- 1/2 cup grated Parmesan cheese
- 2 eggs, beaten
- 2 cups sugar-free marinara sauce
- 1 cup shredded part-skim mozzarella cheese
- Fresh basil leaves (for garnish)
- Cooking spray

Instructions:
1. Preheat oven to 375°F (190°C). Line a baking sheet with parchment paper and lightly grease with cooking spray.
2. In a shallow bowl, combine whole wheat breadcrumbs and grated Parmesan cheese.
3. Dip eggplant slices into beaten eggs, then dredge in breadcrumb mixture, pressing gently to adhere.
4. Place breaded eggplant slices on the prepared baking sheet.

5. Bake for 15-20 minutes, flipping halfway through, until eggplant is golden brown and crispy.
6. Remove from oven and reduce oven temperature to 350°F (175°C).

Fitness Fuel: Zero-Point Recipes

Creating zero-point recipes that fuel an active lifestyle ensures you maintain energy levels without compromising on taste. Here are some recipes including Power Protein Pancakes and Post-Workout Smoothies:

1. Power Protein Pancakes

Ingredients:
- 1 cup rolled oats
- 1 ripe banana
- 1 cup fat-free Greek yogurt
- 2 eggs
- 1 teaspoon baking powder
- 1/2 teaspoon ground cinnamon
- 1/2 teaspoon vanilla extract

- Pinch of salt
- Cooking spray

Instructions:

1. In a blender or food processor, combine rolled oats, ripe banana, fat-free Greek yogurt, eggs, baking powder, ground cinnamon, vanilla extract, and a pinch of salt.
2. Blend until smooth batter forms.
3. Heat a non-stick skillet or griddle over medium heat and lightly coat with cooking spray.
4. Pour pancake batter onto the skillet, using about 1/4 cup for each pancake.
5. Cook until bubbles form on the surface of the pancakes, then flip and cook until golden brown on the other side.
6. Serve warm with fresh fruit, Greek yogurt, or a drizzle of honey.

2. Post-Workout Smoothies

Ingredients:

Berry Blast Smoothie:

- 1 cup mixed berries (strawberries, blueberries, raspberries)
- 1/2 cup fat-free Greek yogurt
- 1 tablespoon chia seeds
- 1/2 cup unsweetened almond milk
- Ice cubes (optional)

Instructions:

1. In a blender, combine mixed berries, fat-free Greek yogurt, chia seeds, unsweetened almond milk, and ice cubes if desired.
2. Blend until smooth and creamy.
3. Pour into a glass and serve immediately.

Green Power Smoothie:

- 1 cup spinach leaves
- 1/2 cup kale leaves, chopped

- 1/2 cucumber, peeled and chopped
- 1/2 avocado, peeled and pitted
- 1 tablespoon fresh ginger, grated
- Juice of 1 lemon
- 1 cup coconut water
- Ice cubes (optional)

Instructions:

1. In a blender, combine spinach leaves, chopped kale leaves, chopped cucumber, peeled and pitted avocado, grated fresh ginger, lemon juice, coconut water, and ice cubes if desired.
2. Blend until smooth and creamy.
3. Pour into a glass and serve immediately.

Banana Peanut Butter Smoothie:

- 1 ripe banana
- 2 tablespoons natural peanut butter
- 1 cup fat-free Greek yogurt
- 1/2 cup unsweetened almond milk
- Ice cubes (optional)

Instructions:

1. In a blender, combine ripe banana, natural peanut butter, fat-free Greek yogurt, unsweetened almond milk, and ice cubes if desired.
2. Blend until smooth and creamy.
3. Pour into a glass and serve immediately.

3. Quinoa Energy Bars

Ingredients:
- 1 cup cooked quinoa, cooled
- 1/2 cup natural almond butter
- 1/4 cup honey or agave syrup
- 1/2 cup rolled oats
- 1/4 cup unsweetened shredded coconut
- 1/4 cup chopped nuts (such as almonds or walnuts)
- 1/4 cup dried fruit (such as cranberries or raisins)
- 1 teaspoon vanilla extract
- Pinch of salt
- Cooking spray

Instructions:
1. Preheat oven to 350°F (175°C). Line an 8x8-inch baking dish with parchment paper and lightly grease with cooking spray.
2. In a large bowl, combine cooked quinoa, natural almond butter, honey or agave syrup, rolled oats, unsweetened shredded coconut, chopped nuts, dried fruit, vanilla extract, and a pinch of salt. Mix well until combined.
3. Transfer mixture to the prepared baking dish, pressing down firmly to flatten evenly.
4. Bake for 20-25 minutes, or until edges are golden brown.
5. Remove from oven and let cool completely in the baking dish.
6. Cut into bars or squares. Store in an airtight container for up to one week.

4. Mediterranean Tuna Salad

Ingredients:
- 2 cans (5 oz each) solid white tuna in water, drained
- 1 cucumber, diced

- 1 bell pepper, diced
- 1/2 red onion, finely chopped
- 1/4 cup Kalamata olives, sliced
- 1/4 cup chopped fresh parsley
- Juice of 1 lemon
- 2 tablespoons olive oil
- Salt and pepper to taste

Instructions:
1. In a large bowl, combine drained solid white tuna, diced cucumber, diced bell pepper, finely chopped red onion, sliced Kalamata olives, and chopped fresh parsley.
2. Drizzle lemon juice and olive oil over the salad ingredients. Toss gently to combine.
3. Season with salt and pepper to taste.
4. Serve chilled as a protein-packed salad.

5. Grilled Chicken Salad with Balsamic Vinaigrette
Ingredients:
- 1 lb boneless, skinless chicken breasts
- Mixed salad greens (such as spinach, arugula, and romaine lettuce)

- Cherry tomatoes, halved
- Cucumber, sliced
- Red onion, thinly sliced
- Balsamic vinaigrette dressing (sugar-free)

Instructions:

1. Preheat grill or grill pan over medium-high heat.
2. Season chicken breasts with salt and pepper.
3. Grill chicken breasts for 6-7 minutes per side, or until cooked through and no longer pink in the center.
4. Remove chicken from grill and let rest for 5 minutes before slicing.
5. In a large bowl, toss mixed salad greens, halved cherry tomatoes, sliced cucumber, and thinly sliced red onion.
6. Divide salad mixture onto plates.
7. Top each salad with sliced grilled chicken breast.
8. Drizzle with balsamic vinaigrette dressing before serving.

These recipes provide a delicious way to maintain a healthy, zero-point diet while supporting an active lifestyle. Adjust ingredients and portions as needed to fit your dietary preferences and nutritional goals.

Budget-Friendly Bites: Economical Zero-Point Meal Ideas

Creating budget-friendly zero-point meal ideas ensures nutritious options without breaking the bank. Here are recipes for Lentil Stew and Chickpea Salad:

1. Lentil Stew

Ingredients:
- 1 cup dried green or brown lentils, rinsed
- 1 onion, chopped
- 2 carrots, chopped
- 2 celery stalks, chopped
- 3 cloves garlic, minced
- 1 can (15 oz) diced tomatoes
- 4 cups low-sodium vegetable broth

- 1 teaspoon ground cumin
- 1/2 teaspoon smoked paprika
- Salt and pepper to taste
- Fresh parsley (for garnish)
- Cooking spray

Instructions:

1. Heat a large pot over medium heat and lightly coat with cooking spray.
2. Add chopped onion, carrots, and celery to the pot. Cook until vegetables are softened, about 5-7 minutes.
3. Stir in minced garlic, ground cumin, and smoked paprika. Cook for an additional minute until fragrant.
4. Add dried lentils, diced tomatoes (with juices), and low-sodium vegetable broth to the pot. Bring to a boil.
5. Reduce heat to low, cover, and simmer for 25-30 minutes, or until lentils are tender.
6. Season with salt and pepper to taste.
7. Serve hot, garnished with fresh parsley.

2. Chickpea Salad

Ingredients:

- 2 cans (15 oz each) chickpeas, rinsed and drained
- 1 cucumber, diced
- 1 bell pepper, diced
- 1/2 red onion, finely chopped
- 1/4 cup chopped fresh parsley
- Juice of 1 lemon
- 2 tablespoons olive oil
- Salt and pepper to taste

Instructions:

1. In a large bowl, combine chickpeas, diced cucumber, diced bell pepper, finely chopped red onion, and chopped fresh parsley.
2. Drizzle lemon juice and olive oil over the salad ingredients. Toss gently to combine.
3. Season with salt and pepper to taste.
4. Serve chilled as a refreshing salad.

3. Vegetable Stir-Fry with Tofu

Ingredients:
- 1 block (14 oz) firm tofu, drained and cubed
- 2 cups mixed vegetables (such as bell peppers, broccoli, and snap peas)
- 1 onion, sliced
- 3 cloves garlic, minced
- 1 tablespoon low-sodium soy sauce
- 1 tablespoon hoisin sauce
- 1 teaspoon sesame oil
- 1/2 teaspoon grated ginger
- Cooked brown rice (optional, for serving)

Instructions:
1. Heat sesame oil in a large skillet or wok over medium-high heat.
2. Add cubed tofu to the skillet, cooking until golden brown on all sides, about 5-7 minutes. Remove tofu from skillet and set aside.
3. In the same skillet, add sliced onion and mixed vegetables. Stir-fry until vegetables are tender-crisp, about 5 minutes.

4. Stir in minced garlic and grated ginger, cooking for an additional minute until fragrant.
5. Return cooked tofu to the skillet.
6. Drizzle low-sodium soy sauce and hoisin sauce over tofu and vegetables, stirring to coat evenly.
7. Cook for 2-3 minutes, or until sauce thickens slightly.
8. Serve hot over cooked brown rice if desired.

4. Zucchini Noodles with Marinara Sauce

Ingredients:
- 4 medium zucchinis, spiralized into noodles
- 2 cups sugar-free marinara sauce
- 1 tablespoon olive oil
- 3 cloves garlic, minced
- Crushed red pepper flakes (optional)
- Fresh basil leaves (for garnish)
- Salt and pepper to taste.

Instructions:

1. Heat olive oil in a large skillet over medium heat.
2. Add minced garlic and crushed red pepper flakes (if using), cooking until garlic is fragrant.
3. Add spiralized zucchini noodles to the skillet. Cook for 2-3 minutes, tossing gently with tongs, until noodles are just tender.
4. Pour sugar-free marinara sauce over zucchini noodles, stirring to coat evenly.
5. Cook for an additional 2-3 minutes, or until sauce is heated through.
6. Season with salt and pepper to taste.
7. Serve hot, garnished with fresh basil leaves.

5. Stuffed Bell Peppers with Quinoa and Black Beans

Ingredients:

- 4 bell peppers, tops cut off and seeds removed
- 1 cup cooked quinoa
- 1 can (15 oz) black beans, rinsed and drained

- 1 cup corn kernels (fresh or frozen)
- 1/2 cup diced tomatoes
- 1 teaspoon ground cumin
- 1/2 teaspoon chili powder
- Salt and pepper to taste
- 1/2 cup shredded reduced-fat cheddar cheese (optional)

Instructions:

1. Preheat oven to 375°F (190°C). Grease a baking dish with cooking spray.
2. In a large bowl, combine cooked quinoa, rinsed black beans, corn kernels, diced tomatoes, ground cumin, chili powder, salt, and pepper.
3. Spoon quinoa mixture evenly into hollowed-out bell peppers.
4. Place stuffed bell peppers upright in the prepared baking dish.
5. Cover dish with foil and bake for 30 minutes.
6. Remove foil and sprinkle shredded reduced-fat cheddar cheese (if using) over the tops of stuffed bell peppers.
7. Bake for an additional 10-15 minutes, or until bell peppers are tender and cheese is melted.

8. Serve hot, garnished with fresh herbs if desired.

These budget-friendly recipes provide tasty and nutritious options for maintaining a healthy, zero-point diet without compromising on flavor. Adjust ingredients and portions as needed to fit your dietary preferences and nutritional goals.

Holiday and Special Occasion Recipes

Creating festive and special occasion recipes that fit into a zero-point diet ensures you can enjoy celebrations while staying healthy. Here are recipes for a Holiday Veggie Platter and Summer Berry Parfait:

1. Holiday Veggie Platter

Ingredients:
- 1 cucumber, sliced
- 1 bell pepper, sliced
- 2 cups cherry tomatoes
- 2 cups snap peas

- 1 cup baby carrots
- 1 cup celery sticks
- Hummus (optional, for dipping)

Instructions:

1. Arrange sliced cucumber, bell pepper, cherry tomatoes, snap peas, baby carrots, and celery sticks on a large serving platter.
2. Serve with hummus for dipping, if desired.
3. Enjoy this colorful and nutritious platter as a festive appetizer or side dish.

2. Summer Berry Parfait

Ingredients:

- 1 cup fat-free Greek yogurt
- 1 cup mixed berries (such as strawberries, blueberries, raspberries)
- 1/4 cup granola (sugar-free)
- Fresh mint leaves (for garnish)

Instructions:

1. In a serving glass or bowl, layer fat-free Greek yogurt, mixed berries, and sugar-free granola.
2. Repeat layers until ingredients are used up, ending with a layer of berries and granola on top.
3. Garnish with fresh mint leaves.
4. Serve immediately as a refreshing and satisfying dessert or breakfast option.

3. Grilled Vegetable Skewers

Ingredients:
- 1 zucchini, sliced into rounds
- 1 yellow squash, sliced into rounds
- 1 red bell pepper, cut into chunks
- 1 yellow bell pepper, cut into chunks
- 1 red onion, cut into chunks
- Cherry tomatoes
- Cooking spray
- Salt and pepper to taste
- Fresh herbs (such as rosemary or thyme, optional)

Instructions:

1. Preheat grill or grill pan over medium-high heat.
2. Thread zucchini rounds, yellow squash rounds, red bell pepper chunks, yellow bell pepper chunks, red onion chunks, and cherry tomatoes onto skewers.
3. Lightly coat skewers with cooking spray and season with salt and pepper.
4. Grill skewers for 8-10 minutes, turning occasionally, until vegetables are tender and lightly charred.
5. Remove from grill and garnish with fresh herbs, if desired.
6. Serve hot as a colorful and flavorful side dish for special occasions.

4. Stuffed Portobello Mushrooms

Ingredients:
- 4 large portobello mushrooms, stems removed
- 1 cup baby spinach, chopped
- 1/2 cup diced tomatoes
- 1/2 cup diced red bell pepper

- 1/4 cup chopped fresh basil
- 1/4 cup shredded reduced-fat mozzarella cheese
- 2 tablespoons balsamic vinegar
- Salt and pepper to taste
- Cooking spray

Instructions:

1. Preheat oven to 375°F (190°C). Line a baking sheet with parchment paper and lightly grease with cooking spray.
2. Place portobello mushrooms on the prepared baking sheet, gill side up.
3. In a medium bowl, combine chopped baby spinach, diced tomatoes, diced red bell pepper, chopped fresh basil, shredded reduced-fat mozzarella cheese, balsamic vinegar, salt, and pepper.
4. Spoon spinach mixture evenly into the hollowed-out portobello mushrooms.
5. Bake for 20-25 minutes, or until mushrooms are tender and filling is heated through.
6. Remove from oven and let cool slightly before serving.

7. Serve warm as a delicious and satisfying main dish or appetizer for special occasions.

5. Fresh Fruit Salad with Citrus Dressing

Ingredients:
- 2 cups mixed fresh fruit (such as strawberries, pineapple, kiwi, and grapes), chopped
- Juice of 1 orange
- Juice of 1 lemon
- 1 tablespoon honey or agave syrup
- Fresh mint leaves (for garnish)

Instructions:
1. In a large bowl, combine mixed fresh fruit.
2. In a small bowl, whisk together orange juice, lemon juice, and honey or agave syrup to make the citrus dressing.
3. Pour citrus dressing over the mixed fruit and gently toss to coat.
4. Garnish with fresh mint leaves.
5. Serve immediately as a light and refreshing dessert or side dish for special occasions.

These recipes offer flavorful options for holidays and special occasions while adhering to a zero-point diet, ensuring you can celebrate without sacrificing health goals. Adjust ingredients and portions as needed to fit your dietary preferences and nutritional goals.

Time-Saving Tips: Quick and Easy Zero-Point Recipes

Creating quick and easy zero-point recipes is essential for busy days. Here are recipes for Instant Pot Chicken Soup and Microwave Steamed Veggies, along with a few more time-saving tips:

1. Instant Pot Chicken Soup
Ingredients:
- 1 lb boneless, skinless chicken breasts
- 4 cups low-sodium chicken broth
- 2 carrots, sliced
- 2 celery stalks, sliced

- 1 onion, chopped
- 3 cloves garlic, minced
- 1 teaspoon dried thyme
- 1 teaspoon dried rosemary
- Salt and pepper to taste
- Cooking spray

Instructions:

1. Lightly coat the bottom of the Instant Pot with cooking spray. Set to sauté mode.
2. Add chopped onion and minced garlic, cooking until softened, about 2-3 minutes.
3. Add boneless, skinless chicken breasts to the Instant Pot, cooking until lightly browned on all sides.
4. Add sliced carrots, sliced celery stalks, dried thyme, dried rosemary, salt, and pepper to the Instant Pot.
5. Pour low-sodium chicken broth over the ingredients in the Instant Pot.
6. Close and lock the lid. Set the Instant Pot to manual high pressure for 10 minutes.

7. Once cooking is complete, allow natural pressure release for 5 minutes, then quick release any remaining pressure.
8. Open the lid carefully. Remove chicken breasts from the Instant Pot and shred with two forks.
9. Return shredded chicken to the Instant Pot and stir to combine.
10. Serve hot, garnished with fresh herbs if desired.

2. Microwave Steamed Veggies

Ingredients:
- 2 cups mixed vegetables (such as broccoli florets, cauliflower florets, and carrot slices)
- 2 tablespoons water
- Salt and pepper to taste

Instructions:
1. Place mixed vegetables in a microwave-safe bowl.
2. Add water to the bowl.

3. Cover the bowl with a microwave-safe lid or microwave-safe plastic wrap, leaving a small vent.
4. Microwave on high for 3-4 minutes, or until vegetables are tender-crisp.
5. Carefully remove from microwave and drain any excess water.
6. Season with salt and pepper to taste.
7. Serve hot as a quick and nutritious side dish.

3. Turkey and Bean Chili

Ingredients:
- 1 lb ground turkey
- 1 onion, chopped
- 1 bell pepper, chopped
- 2 cloves garlic, minced
- 1 can (15 oz) black beans, rinsed and drained
- 1 can (15 oz) kidney beans, rinsed and drained
- 1 can (15 oz) diced tomatoes
- 2 cups low-sodium chicken broth
- 2 tablespoons chili powder

- 1 teaspoon ground cumin
- Salt and pepper to taste
- Cooking spray

Instructions:

1. Heat a large pot over medium heat and lightly coat with cooking spray.
2. Add chopped onion, chopped bell pepper, and minced garlic to the pot. Cook until vegetables are softened, about 5-7 minutes.
3. Add ground turkey to the pot, cooking until browned and cooked through.
4. Stir in black beans, kidney beans, diced tomatoes (with juices), low-sodium chicken broth, chili powder, ground cumin, salt, and pepper.
5. Bring chili to a boil, then reduce heat to low. Simmer uncovered for 20-25 minutes, stirring occasionally.
6. Adjust seasoning with salt and pepper to taste before serving.
7. Serve hot, garnished with chopped green onions or shredded reduced-fat cheese if desired.

4. Tuna Salad Lettuce Wraps

Ingredients:
- 2 cans (5 oz each) solid white tuna in water, drained
- 1/2 cup fat-free Greek yogurt
- 1/4 cup diced celery
- 1/4 cup diced red onion
- 1 tablespoon lemon juice
- Salt and pepper to taste
- Romaine lettuce leaves (for serving)

Instructions:
1. In a medium bowl, combine drained solid white tuna, fat-free Greek yogurt, diced celery, diced red onion, lemon juice, salt, and pepper.
2. Mix until well combined.
3. Spoon tuna salad mixture onto individual romaine lettuce leaves.
4. Roll up lettuce leaves to form wraps.
5. Serve immediately as a quick and protein-packed lunch or snack.

5. Eggplant Caprese Salad

Ingredients:
- 1 large eggplant, sliced into rounds
- 2 tomatoes, sliced
- 1/2 cup fresh mozzarella, sliced
- Fresh basil leaves
- Balsamic vinegar
- Salt and pepper to taste
- Cooking spray

Instructions:
1. Preheat grill or grill pan over medium-high heat. Lightly coat eggplant rounds with cooking spray.
2. Grill eggplant rounds for 3-4 minutes per side, or until tender and lightly charred.
3. Remove from grill and let cool slightly.
4. On a serving platter, layer grilled eggplant rounds, tomato slices, and fresh mozzarella slices.
5. Top with fresh basil leaves.
6. Drizzle with balsamic vinegar.
7. Season with salt and pepper to taste.

8. Serve warm or at room temperature as a flavorful and satisfying appetizer or side dish.

These recipes and tips provide quick and easy ways to prepare delicious zero-point meals on busy days. Adjust ingredients and portions as needed to fit your dietary preferences and nutritional goals.

Mindful Eating: Strategies for Enjoying Zero-Point Foods

Here are recipes for Slow-Cooked Ratatouille and Savor-the-Moment Salad, along with mindful eating strategies for your new book:

1. Slow-Cooked Ratatouille

Ingredients:
- 1 eggplant, diced
- 2 zucchinis, diced
- 1 yellow squash, diced
- 1 red bell pepper, diced
- 1 yellow bell pepper, diced

- 1 onion, chopped
- 3 cloves garlic, minced
- 1 can (15 oz) diced tomatoes
- 2 tablespoons tomato paste
- 1 teaspoon dried thyme
- 1 teaspoon dried oregano
- Salt and pepper to taste
- Fresh basil leaves (for garnish)
- Cooking spray

Instructions:

1. Lightly coat a slow cooker with cooking spray.
2. Layer diced eggplant, diced zucchinis, diced yellow squash, diced red bell pepper, diced yellow bell pepper, chopped onion, and minced garlic in the slow cooker.
3. In a small bowl, mix diced tomatoes, tomato paste, dried thyme, dried oregano, salt, and pepper. Pour mixture over vegetables in the slow cooker, stirring gently to combine.
4. Cover and cook on low heat for 6-8 hours, or until vegetables are tender.

5. Adjust seasoning with salt and pepper to taste before serving.
6. Serve hot, garnished with fresh basil leaves.

2. Savor-the-Moment Salad

Ingredients:
- 4 cups mixed greens (such as spinach, arugula, and kale)
- 1 cup cherry tomatoes, halved
- 1 cucumber, sliced
- 1/2 red onion, thinly sliced
- 1/4 cup sliced almonds, toasted
- 1/4 cup crumbled feta cheese (optional)
- Balsamic vinaigrette or lemon olive oil dressing (to taste)
- Salt and pepper to taste

Instructions:
1. In a large salad bowl, combine mixed greens, halved cherry tomatoes, sliced cucumber, thinly sliced red onion, toasted sliced almonds, and crumbled feta cheese (if using).

2. Drizzle with balsamic vinaigrette or lemon olive oil dressing.

3. Toss gently to coat ingredients evenly.

4. Season with salt and pepper to taste.

5. Serve immediately as a refreshing and nutritious salad.

3. Lemon Garlic Shrimp with Quinoa

Ingredients:
- 1 lb large shrimp, peeled and deveined
- 1 cup quinoa, rinsed
- 2 cups low-sodium chicken broth
- 3 tablespoons olive oil
- 3 cloves garlic, minced
- Juice of 1 lemon
- 1 teaspoon lemon zest
- Salt and pepper to taste
- Fresh parsley (for garnish)

Instructions:
1. In a medium saucepan, heat 1 tablespoon olive oil over medium heat.

2. Add minced garlic and cook until fragrant, about 1 minute.

3. Stir in quinoa and cook for an additional 2 minutes, stirring frequently.

4. Pour low-sodium chicken broth over the quinoa mixture. Bring to a boil.

5. Reduce heat to low, cover, and simmer for 15-20 minutes, or until quinoa is cooked and liquid is absorbed.

6. In a large skillet, heat remaining 2 tablespoons olive oil over medium-high heat.

7. Add peeled and deveined shrimp to the skillet. Cook shrimp until pink and opaque, about 2-3 minutes per side.

8. Stir in lemon juice, lemon zest, salt, and pepper.

9. Serve lemon garlic shrimp over cooked quinoa.

10. Garnish with fresh parsley before serving.

4. Cauliflower Fried Rice
Ingredients:
- 1 head cauliflower, grated (or 4 cups cauliflower rice)

- 1 cup frozen peas and carrots, thawed
- 2 eggs, beaten
- 3 tablespoons low-sodium soy sauce
- 1 tablespoon sesame oil
- 2 cloves garlic, minced
- 1/2 cup chopped green onions
- Salt and pepper to taste
- Cooking spray

Instructions:

1. Heat a large skillet or wok over medium heat and lightly coat with cooking spray.
2. Add minced garlic and chopped green onions to the skillet, cooking until softened, about 2-3 minutes.
3. Push garlic and green onions to one side of the skillet. Pour beaten eggs into the empty side of the skillet.
4. Scramble eggs until fully cooked, breaking into small pieces with a spatula.
5. Stir in grated cauliflower (or cauliflower rice) and thawed frozen peas and carrots.

6. Drizzle low-sodium soy sauce and sesame oil over the cauliflower mixture, tossing to combine evenly.
7. Cook for 5-7 minutes, stirring frequently, until cauliflower rice is tender and heated through.
8. Season with salt and pepper to taste.
9. Serve hot as a nutritious and flavorful alternative to traditional fried rice.

5. Greek Yogurt Chicken Salad

Ingredients:
- 2 cups shredded cooked chicken breast
- 1/2 cup fat-free Greek yogurt
- 1/4 cup diced celery
- 1/4 cup diced red onion
- 1/4 cup halved grapes
- 1 tablespoon lemon juice
- Salt and pepper to taste
- Lettuce leaves or whole-grain bread (for serving).

Instructions:
1. In a medium bowl, combine shredded cooked chicken breast, fat-free Greek yogurt, diced celery, diced red onion, halved grapes, lemon juice, salt, and pepper.
2. Mix until well combined.
3. Serve chicken salad on lettuce leaves as a light and satisfying meal or as a sandwich filling with whole-grain bread.

These recipes and mindful eating strategies encourage enjoying zero-point foods while savoring flavors and maintaining a healthy lifestyle. Adjust ingredients and portions as needed to fit your dietary preferences and nutritional goals.

Conclusion: Embracing Zero-Point Wonders

Congratulations on embarking on a journey towards a healthier lifestyle with "Zero Point Wonders: The Ultimate Weight Loss Cookbook." Throughout this book, we've explored the incredible benefits of zero-point eating and discovered how simple, yet delicious, recipes can transform our approach to food and wellness.

Recap of the Benefits

Zero-point foods offer more than just a way to manage weight—they provide a foundation for a balanced and nutritious diet. By focusing on these foods, you've empowered yourself with options that are satisfying, nutrient-dense, and naturally low in calories. From vibrant salads to hearty soups and flavorful main dishes, each recipe in this book has been crafted to not only tantalize your taste buds but also support your health goals.

Encouragement to Continue the Journey

As you continue your journey, remember that every meal is an opportunity to nourish your body and delight your senses. Whether you're preparing a quick lunch for one or hosting a gathering with friends and family, these recipes are designed to fit seamlessly into your lifestyle. Embrace mindful eating practices, savor each bite, and celebrate the positive changes you're making.

Gratitude

I want to extend my heartfelt gratitude for choosing "**Zero Point Wonders**" as your companion in this transformative journey. Your commitment to health and well-being inspires me, and I hope these recipes bring joy and success to your kitchen.

Stay Connected

For ongoing support and inspiration, connect with us online and share your experiences. Together, we can continue to explore the endless possibilities of zero-point eating and celebrate the joys of a healthier, more vibrant life.

**Here's to Your Health!
With warmest regards,**

[Victor C. Sell]

This conclusion summarizes the benefits of zero-point eating while encouraging readers to embrace a healthier lifestyle with gratitude and optimism. Adjust the message to resonate with your personal voice and the overall tone of your book.

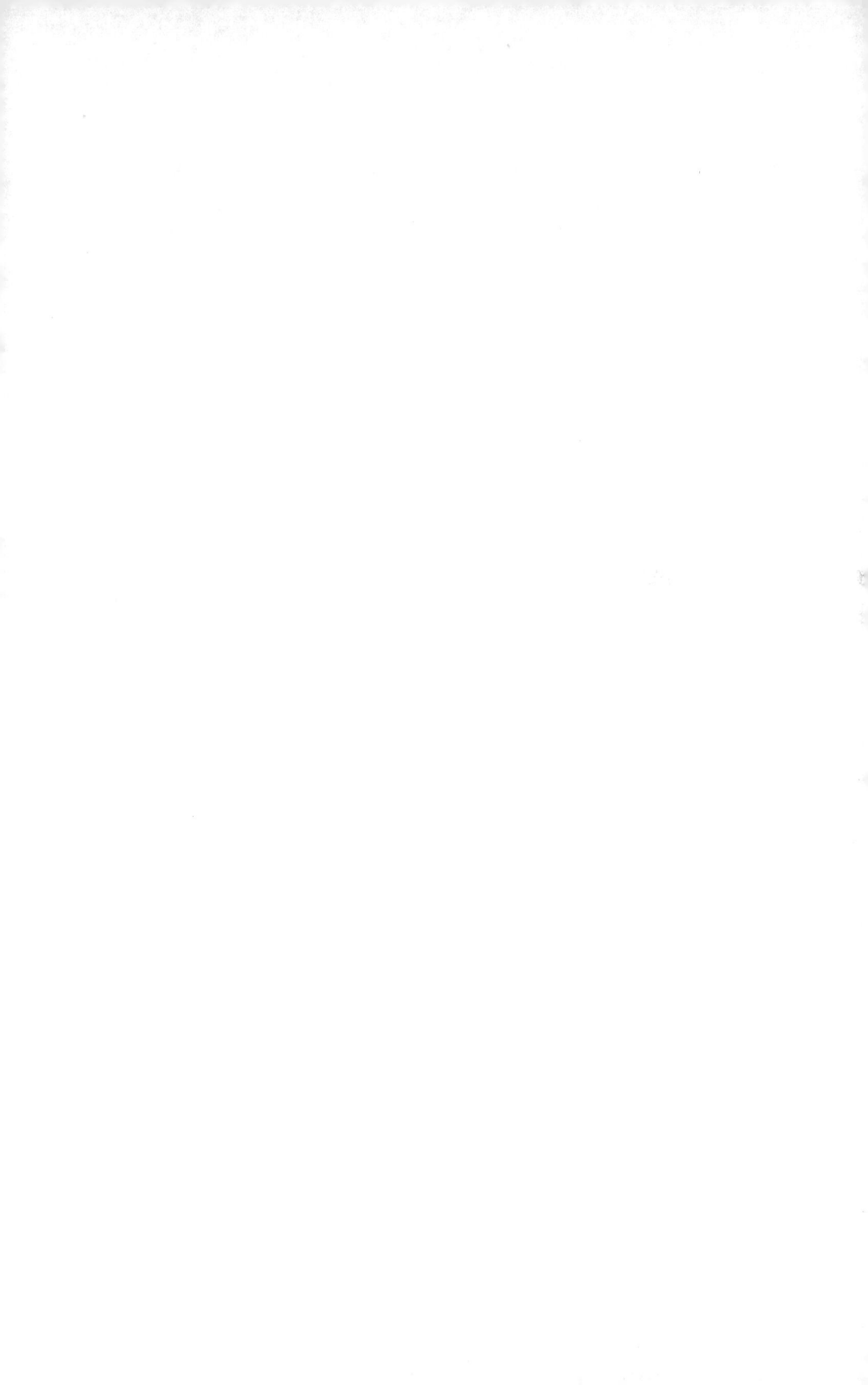

Made in the USA
Middletown, DE
20 July 2024